Dr. Sabrina Morgen

MANIPULATION *Under*
ANESTHESIA

*Rediscovering an Effective, Safe, Non-Surgical,
Non-Invasive, Pain Relieving Procedure*

All rights reserved under the international and American copyright conventions.
First published in the United States of America.

ISBN: 1460970691
ISBN-13: 9781460970690
Library of Congress Control Number: 2011903772
CreateSpace, Charleston, South Carolina

⌇

About the Author

Dr. Sabrina Morgen is the clinic director of Physicians Wellness Care, Inc., and has been in private practice since 1998. She received her Doctorate of Chiropractic from the Los Angeles College of Chiropractic in 1997. Having performed thousands of MUA's in various outpatient ambulatory surgery centers in Palm Beach, Broward, and Indian River County, Dr. Morgen has helped many patients alleviate pain and suffering while improving their quality of life.

Dr. Morgen is a chiropractic physician who received her MUA certification in 2006, and is certified as a neuropathy doctor as well as a dual Fellow in acupuncture and integrative cancer therapy. Initially, she experienced trepidation toward the MUA procedure, understanding that some DCs may wonder why anesthesia is necessary to perform an adjustment. After further research and speaking to the patients prior to and post MUA, she learned that she could do more to help them. Some patients are unable to "hold" their adjustments and others have had too much damage to their musculoskeletal structure, so by placing them under twilight sedation, this allows them to receive the benefits of joint mobilization without resistance. The bottom line is to do what serves the patient best.

Offering MUA as an option when other conservative treatments have failed is a wonderful alternative to surgery. This allows physicians to keep Hippocrates' oath, which is: "First, do no harm."

❦

Introduction

FACT: Chronic back pain affects between 75 and 90 percent of the population at some point in their lives.

Chronic back pain is "a major health-care issue," according to Xuemei Luo, Ph.D., Duke University Medical Center.

Conservative, conventional treatments for back pain, as well as for chronic neck pain, often fail. After weeks, months, or even years of treatments, some individuals are unwilling or unqualified due to age, weight, or other medical conditions to undergo surgery. Others are frightened of long-term use of over-the-counter and prescription medications.

For these individuals, there is an alternative treatment. While treatment involves outpatient status at either an ambulatory surgical center or a hospital, it involves no surgery and no invasive methods.

The procedure is called manipulation under anesthesia (MUA) and is a non-invasive therapy that has been utilized successfully for nearly a century to help people overcome pain, discomfort, and limited range of motion.

MUA is a variation of the standard in-office manipulation in which a chiropractic doctor uses his or her hands to physically adjust the spine in order to achieve the maximum level of pain relief.

Manipulation under anesthesia is truly an appropriate name. In this specific procedure, the patient is placed under a mild anesthesia, sometimes referred to as "twilight" or mild sedation. Then the professional team, usually an osteopath and a chiropractic physician, adjusts and stretches the patient's particular area of concern, which may include the spine, ankles, and other extremities, such as shoulders, arms, legs, knees, elbows, pelvis, and/or hips. The application of these movements normally would be too painful to consider or apply under the patient's specific condition(s) without sedation.

When the MUA procedure is combined with simple follow-up therapies, this procedure not only eliminates the patient's pain, but also restores or vastly improves the patient's range of motion. The benefits, however, are not limited to just chronic neck and back conditions.

Individuals have found that this type of treatment is an effective and safe alternative to conventional treatment for the following health conditions:

- fibromyalgia
- frozen shoulder
- sciatica (where disc bulges are contained less than five millimeters)
- low-back and neck pain
- neuralgia
- radiculitis
- headaches/migraine syndrome
- TMJ (Costen's syndrome)
- RSD (reflex sympathetic dystrophy)
- cervical and lumbar disc conditions
- joint calcification
- capsulitis of the hip
- torticollis
- carpal tunnel syndrome
- piriformis syndrome
- pelvic instability
- gait abnormality imbalance
- curvature of the spine
- stiff knee syndrome
- conditions where narcotics are of little benefit

MUA, the procedure, is supported by scientific clinical research. Results of one study, for example, published several years ago in the *Journal of Manipulative and Physiological Therapeutics*, revealed a significantly high success rate. The research investigated a group of patients whose conditions had not improved despite months of in-office chiropractic care and physical therapy.

All individuals in this study underwent manipulation under anesthesia. As part of the research, a quality assurance review was conducted afterward. This review discovered that 70 percent of the people interviewed following the procedure reported that they were "very satisfied" with the level of improvements.

Another study was recently conducted to evaluate the changes in the level of pain and the extent of disability for those individuals who suffered from chronic back pain. The study involved two patient groups.

Both groups received an initial four- to six-week series of conservative in-office manipulation and physical therapy. Following this, one group received MUA while the other continued with the typical in-office procedure. The researchers collected follow-up data at six-week, three-month, six-month, and one-year intervals.

Nearly 66 percent of those undergoing the MUA reported significant improvements in the level of their pain and the extent of their disability at the three-month mark. At the one-year mark, a full 64 percent had reported that they have maintained that level of pain relief and renewed mobility.

Unfortunately, many people, including medical professionals, haven't heard of this particular procedure. But that doesn't mean it's new—because it's not! In fact, MUA has been an established procedure since the 1930s. This procedure was first used by osteopathic physicians, as well as orthopedic surgeons, for many years as a proven form of treatment.

The first documentation of MUA in the United States was in 1948 in the *Journal of American Osteopath Association*. In summary, the article reported that the success rate was between 80 and 90 percent—just about the same that the procedure produces today.

The distinguished and well-respected British medical journal *Lancet* published what's thought to be the earliest clinical study on manipulation under anesthesia in the 1930s. This study overall uncovered that 75 percent of the individuals who underwent the MUA procedure showed distinct improvements.

Doctors of osteopathy have been performing manipulation under anesthesia intermittently throughout the 1950s and 1960s. In the 1970s and 1980s, MUA wasn't utilized much as a treatment. But a group of progressive chiropractic doctors in Texas resurrected it in the 1980s. That's when MUA began to garner the recognition that it has today. Manipulation under anesthesia is an established medical procedure with a CPT Code designation of 22505, as noted in the *American Medical Association's Current Procedural Terminology Publication*.

By the end of the 1980s, a group of doctors created an adjusting protocol. They had established a series of manipulations that worked best for certain types of pains and locations of discomfort, and had also concluded that the greatest benefits were gained when three consecutive treatments were applied.

During this last decade, manipulation under anesthesia has again enjoyed a renewed popularity. And rightly so! The tremendous advances in anesthesiology have contributed greatly to this remarkably effective technique.

In fact, in 1995, a group of physicians from several disciplines formed the National Academy of MUA Physicians, which finally developed formal national standards and protocols for the manipulation under anesthesia procedure. These guidelines have now been universally accepted.

The National Academy of MUA Physicians is continually updating the standards and protocols in order to provide patients with the highest quality of care.

Chapter 1:

෧෨

What Is Manipulation under Anesthesia?

To fully understand manipulation under anesthesia (MUA), you need to have a full knowledge of the general concepts that undergird biomechanics of the body. The MUA treatment is based on the idea that the underlying cause of pain is the restricted movement of the spine and joints, and shortening of attached muscles. The restricted movement leads to the reduced function one experiences.

Manipulation—which involves physically adjusting the spinal column, joint, or extremity—seeks to restore full spinal and joint movement, and, in turn, improves the function of the area as well as alleviates the pain.

It doesn't take a major injury or a traumatic event to restrict spinal movement. Poor, inadequate, or even incorrect function of the spine can be an irritant to vital nerves in the spine. The spine controls not only posture but much of the overall movement of the body. The stress from the restriction of spinal and joint movement causes discomfort and pain.

Patients often undergo various treatments, such as physical therapy, chiropractic care, epidural injections, back surgery, or other treatments, that do not address scar tissue or fibrous adhesions. Some patients feel temporarily better with these treatments, but their pain often returns.

Manipulation: A Hands-On Approach to Health

Chiropractors use their hands in applying a gentle, sudden—but very controlled—force to a joint in order to realign it to its natural, proper position. As a result of manipulation, one often hears a cracking sound, called "cavitation," made by the separation of the joint surfaces.

Manipulation allows the body's innate healing processes to work. For most patients, this is enough to help relieve the discomfort, restore range of motion in the subject area, and provide full function. But for all the good the manipulation provides for the patients, we're still left with the question of why manipulation works in the first place.

Some experts believe that manipulation of the joints stimulates joint movement receptors. Receptors are your body's position sensors that communicate to the brain the location of the joint.

The stimulation affects the way the entire nervous system performs. Depending on the location of the nerve irritation, one may display symptoms of pain in different areas of the body. That's why manipulation is successful for a wide variety of problems, such as headaches and abdominal pain, as well as shoulder, arm, and wrist conditions.

There are instances, though, when the pain is so severe and movement is so restricted that conservative manipulation is not effective. The challenge for the chiropractor is then to provide full manipulation of the subject areas without causing an enormous amount of pain for the patient.

Before we discuss the procedure itself, we need to discuss the "anesthesia" portion. One should not confuse it with the amount, type, and strength of anesthetics one would receive from back surgery or any other kind of invasive surgery. During surgery, one is completely unconscious for hours.

With MUA, one is not exposed to the potential dangers of general anesthetic. An intravenous sedative is administered by a board-certified anesthesiologist. The patient is conscious enough to preserve protective reflexes. The sedation lasts for fifteen to twenty minutes, at most. Typically, Diprivan and/or Versed are utilized.

While under this "twilight" anesthesia and some sedation, the body gains the benefit of a greater range of manipulation, becoming more compliant and flexible.

If the patient is fully conscious during this procedure, the doctor could only perform limited manipulations. If you have undergone in-office manipulation before, then you can relate readily to the limitations of receiving manipulations when you're under chronic, stubborn, and severe pain.

The level of pain the patient is experiencing limits the range of the manipulation during an in-office visit. The body's natural reflexes are to react to any attempt to stretch the muscles, joints, tendons, and related parts of the body because it hurts. However, with manipulation under anesthesia, the patient's body isn't resisting the manipulation because the patient does not feel the pain.

The stretches and manipulations that the doctor performs during MUA actually release fibrous adhesions and scar tissue around the patient's spine, extremities, and the surrounding soft tissue, which are directly responsible for the chronic pain.

In fact, the important role that the anesthetic plays in this procedure cannot be overemphasized. When the patient undergoes this therapy, he or she is lightly sedated; the muscle spasm cycle literally shuts off. This allows for a wider range of spinal and joint movement.

The anesthetic provides for complete muscle relaxation. This means the patient's shortened muscles, which are the ones causing the discomfort, pain, and limited range of motion, can be stretched beyond the point where the pain is consciously tolerable. This, in turn, releases the adhesions caused by the scar tissue.

Finally, the sedation provides much needed relief to the nerves in the joints and muscles since they have been the recipients of the pain and have been irritated because of the condition of the spine and joints.

A Team Approach to MUA

Unlike in-office manipulation, which requires the skill of one chiropractor, MUA entails the involvement of a team of medical specialists. Not only will the patient's doctor be there to perform the manipulation, but the patient's doctor will be accompanied by a trained and licensed osteopath physician as well as another chiropractic physician who is certified in manipulation under anesthesia.

And, of course, the patient is being monitored throughout the procedure by a board-certified anesthesiologist. In fact, a complete anesthesia record is maintained throughout this procedure and the patient's blood pressure is carefully checked. Readings are obtained about every five minutes.

To gain the full effects of this treatment, the patient's health care provider may recommend that the patient undergo three consecutive days of treatment. Studies indicate that this provides the most benefits.

Depending upon the status of the condition, the severity of the pain, and the judgment of the doctor, the patient may undergo a single session of MUA or up to a series of three. In some rare instances, the patient's doctor may recommend up to five consecutive sessions.

The majority of doctors believe that to achieve pain relief and maximum functional restoration to the spine, three treatments are necessary. This is especially true, they contend, if the health condition involves the presence of chronic fibrosis, or scar tissue due to injury or inflammation, and injury to a disc.

Most physicians who practice MUA believe that the serial approach may be the gentlest and safest practice to fully restore a patient's range of motion. According to Timothy Mills, D.C., writing in the publication *Dynamic Chiropractic,* "the serial application [of MUA] has a greater safety factor than a single application when the clinical goal is to fully restore…range of motion in cases of periarticular or articular fibrosis."

He further states: "There appears to be a cumulative effect added to the first application…especially when major muscle groups, such as the hamstring, pelvic and paravertebral musculature, are stretched gradually in series."

There are also two more advantages to the series approach. The physician is able to be more specific when restoring spinal function, and the doctor is able to better monitor the approach when performing the treatment. When performed in this manner, the doctor can achieve the very best possible maximum clinical benefits.

The serial approach, moreover, takes into consideration the state of the intervertebral tissue. Despite the fact that the patient is anesthetized, the fibrotic muscles, as well as the other soft tissue that is scarred, do not automatically become elastic. Repeating the application over a three-day period allows for an increased amount of stretching with each application.

In this regard, Mills quotes G.D. Maitland, in his book *Vertebral Manipulation:* "Rather than trying to achieve a full range of movement in one manipulation, it is often better to manipulate more gently on two or more occasions."

The Goals of MUA

The ultimate goals of manipulation under anesthesia are to:

- Allow complete muscle relaxation so that the doctor can eliminate and/or release the scar tissue (adhesions) that has formed in and around the joints as well as in the muscles.
- Stretch and lengthen persistent shortened muscles, ligaments, and tendons.
- Eliminate and/or relieve the chronic pain as well as the radiating symptoms caused by the damaged intervertebral discs and scarred soft tissue. Some disc injuries are serious enough to require surgery, but these types of injuries are relatively infrequent.
- Interrupt the cycle of chronic muscle spasm to allow for increased movement.
- Sedate the pain-perceiving nerves that have been irritated due to the dysfunctional spine or joint.
- Decrease chronic muscle spasm.
- Overcome super-sensitivity of injured areas, making the patient unable to cooperate for effective treatment.

MUA is not an invasive surgery, and the procedure is very gentle. An intravenous catheter is inserted into the patient's arm and a small amount of anesthesia is administered by a board-certified anesthesiologist. The anesthesia wears off in about thirty minutes. While the anesthesia is light and wears off quickly, the patient's doctor requires that someone accompany the patient home. (Most centers provide transportation upon request.)

The procedure itself takes no longer than thirty minutes. Usually the professionals can complete MUA within fifteen to twenty minutes.

Following the completion of MUA, the patient is taken into a recovery room. Medical personnel will carefully monitor the patient, who will be given supplemental oxygen according to the protocol of the clinic or hospital.

Chapter 2:

༄

The Benefits of Manipulation under Anesthesia

"MUA is recommended," according to Thomas Dorman, M.D. and orthopedist, in *Diagnosis Technique in Orthopedic Medicine,* "when the patient has failed at conservative in-office care."

This being said, the doctor will not consider the patient as a candidate for MUA until the patient has undergone a minimum of six to eight weeks of conservative therapy. This could be in the form of medical treatment via pain-killing prescription drugs, chiropractic care, or physical therapy.

MUA has been proven to provide effective relief for individuals who have experienced a wide range of various conditions, from chronic back pain to fibromyalgia.

Low-Back Pain

Perhaps the largest group of individuals who may benefit from manipulation under anesthesia consists of those suffering from chronic low-back pain. In fact, according to some medical experts, low-back pain is "the most expensive benign [medical] condition in industrialized countries. It is, by far, the most common cause of physical limitations in people who are younger than forty-five years of age."

Medically, chronic low-back pain is defined as a pain that lasts longer than three months. For many individuals, low-back pain is caused by a degenerative condition, events normally associated with wear and tear of the body and the aging process, or a traumatic event to the spine.

However, there are other causes of chronic low-back pain. Fibrositis, which is the accumulation of scar tissue on the muscle, inflammatory spondyloarthropathy, a chronic disease of the joints, and various metabolic bone conditions can also cause chronic low-back pain. Additionally, back pain can be caused by sciatica, as well as disc herniation and protrusion or a bulging of the disc.

Perhaps the most frustrating aspect of this medical condition, however, is when the doctor cannot find the physical cause of the pain. In this case, it is not uncommon for both the physician and the patient to question the pain's origin.

The extent of how back pain affects society is staggering. Each year, between 5 and 20 percent of Americans complain of back pain in some form. In Europe, that statistic hovers between 25 and 45 percent. Low-back pain, moreover, accounts for nearly 20 percent of all workers' compensation claims in the United States.

Additionally, this high rate of frequency costs the United States in a variety of ways, between lost productivity and the costs of treatment. It is estimated conservatively that it costs the US $85 million dollars yearly.

Even after a Decade of Back Pain, Relief Is Possible

Some individuals have suffered for a decade or more with back pain that has been unresponsive to conservative care.

One study examined individuals who had been plagued with back pain for ten years. Imagine an entire decade of enduring chronic pain, day in and day out, until they discovered manipulation under anesthesia. Statistics show that 87 percent of these individuals, who thought absolutely nothing would take away their stubborn pain, reported a remarkable improvement in their symptoms.

Another study examined intractable pain that plagued individuals for up to eighteen years. Two researchers followed one hundred and seventy-one patients whose pain varied in length from several months to eighteen years. In each of these cases, conventional, conservative therapy proved unsuccessful.

The results of MUA were remarkable, especially considering the amount of time some of the patients had endured their particular condition. More than half of the individuals indicated that their pain had improved greatly.

Another 20 percent said that their pain was relieved somewhat and a full one-quarter of the recipients of MUA said that their long-standing pain had completely disappeared.

That means that 95 percent experienced some type of relief that had been eluding them, in some cases for up to two decades. Imagine, after nearly twenty years of fighting off constant pain, to be able to call a truce!

Cervical and Thoracic Pain Relieved by MUA

Low-back pain is an epidemic. However, individuals who suffer from neck and mid-back pain, medically described as cervical and thoracic pain, respectively, can also benefit from MUA. A recent study indicates MUA provided a significant improvement for these conditions.

Individuals who had experienced no relief from their cervical, thoracic, or lumbar pain with conservative therapy were treated with a series of three sessions of manipulation under anesthesia. They were also provided with four to six weeks of follow-up therapies. Another group received continued conventional manipulation.

Of those who received the MUA, more than 50 percent reported substantial improvement in their condition, compared to just 25 percent of those who received the conventional treatment.

Herniated Disc

There are several signs that may indicate that your back pain is due to a herniated disc. Symptoms of this condition include having a difficult time with ordinary movement, whether it is bending or simply sitting. A sharp pain in your back radiating into one of your legs may also indicate the presence of a herniated disc. The only comfortable position you may find is lying on your back.

A herniated disc is one that has ruptured. Your discs are located between the vertebrae of your spine, where they serve as cushions. They prevent the hard, bony vertebrae from making contact with each other.

A disc is composed of an outer ring of fibrous tissue with a gel-like substance in the center. With a composition of nearly 80 percent water, it has no blood supply of its own. This means that as you age, the center of the disc becomes firm and eventually begins to dry out. In fact, this dessication process begins while you are still in your thirties. By the time most people reach fifty, the center or nucleus is dry and fibrous, and merges with the outer ring of the disc.

With time, the outer portion of the disc becomes prone to tearing. As a result, the nucleus or center may emerge through this hole, causing a rupture or, as it is frequently called, a "herniation." If this center extrudes far enough, it can irritate the closest nerve, causing the pain in your back.

Before the rupture of the disc, you may feel at least one episode, and sometimes multiple episodes, of acute low-back pain. Once it has fully ruptured, the primary symptom then becomes a sharp or throbbing pain in your back, accompanied by a shooting pain down the leg.

If the herniated disc is in the middle or lower portion of your back, you may also feel a weakness, tingling, or even numbness in your buttocks, legs, or feet. A shooting pain that occurs when you cough, sneeze, or even strain may also indicate a herniated disc.

Many people are failed by conventional medical treatment. Others do not want to expose themselves to long-term use of either over-the-counter or prescription medications. Others have found that because of the severity of the pain, in-office physical therapy and chiropractic manipulation has been temporary.

Many discover that MUA helps when no other treatments can. A series of applications of this procedure has proven successful for those who have tolerated the pain, discomfort, and limited range of motion of herniated discs for months and years.

Chronic Neck Pain

Harvard Medical School found that seven out of ten individuals will experience neck pain sometime during their lifetime. Neck pain is common, according to the experts at Harvard, because the neck is not only supporting the heavy weight of the head, but also performing the tasks of tilting, turning, and nodding the skull.

It is not unusual that, after years of normal use, overuse, and sometimes even misuse, pain in the neck develops.

Just as with chronic low-back pain, neck pain has many possible causes. If your pain radiates into your arm and even to your hands and fingers, you may have a cervical herniated disc or foraminal stenosis (the narrowing of the spinal canal through which the nerves travel), pinching a nerve in the neck.

This pain, additionally, may be accompanied by a tingling or numbness in your arms or hands. For some people, this develops suddenly; for others, it's a gradual onset.

If your pain is caused by cervical foraminal stenosis, then it might be related to certain activities or positions. This particular condition is normally accepted as part of the normal age-related changes of the joints of the neck.

If your pain, in addition to radiating down your arm, also produces a lack of coordination in the arms and legs, along with difficulty in performing the finer motor skills, then it could be caused by cervical stenosis with myelopathy. The term "myelopathy" refers to the dysfunction of the spinal cord itself.

For some individuals, conditions with the neck are not alleviated by either conventional medical treatment or through conservative chiropractic manipulation. Many, though, have discovered that MUA is a safe and effective approach to alleviating their condition.

Fibromyalgia

Fibromyalgia is a chronic condition characterized by an unspecific pain in your muscles, ligaments, and tendons. Other symptoms of this health condition include trigger points in the body that are tender to the touch without any apparent cause.

Also associated with this disorder is a fatigue that reaches, according to many who are afflicted with it, into your very soul.

Fibromyalgia is a very difficult condition for doctors to diagnose. Not only do the symptoms of fibromyalgia differ from one individual to the next, but even with the same individual, the symptoms may fluctuate from day to day. External factors, such as the weather, the level of stress you are experiencing, and the amount of physical activity you are performing, affect your symptoms.

If you experience chronic pain, have eleven out of eighteen specific trigger points, and have a decrease in serotonin levels with exhaustive fatigue, you may have fibromyalgia. Other indications of this disorder also include recurrent headaches as well as experiencing TMJ (temporomandibular joint) pain.

Conventional medical treatment offers little in the way of effectiveness for this disorder. However, manipulation under anesthesia has helped many individuals who had suffered for months or years with fibromyalgia.

Myofascitis

You may also be a candidate for MUA if you suffer from myofascitis. This is the inflammation of a muscle as well as its fascia, the strong connective tissue around the muscle. The fascia performs several duties, including enveloping and isolating the muscles of your body. It does this in order to provide a form of structural support and protection. One of the causes of this inflammation is micro-trauma, damage caused by a repetitive motion. It is not unusual for those who lift weights to acquire this inflammation.

Fibrous Adhesions

Fibrous adhesions are scar tissue in the muscle, which may occur as a result of myofascitis, the inflammation of the muscle and its connective tissue. Many times fibrous adhesion develops following a surgery and in those who suffer from chronic pain. However fibrous adhesions develop, this scar tissue limits the range of motion of the muscle and joints. This is a very painful condition that MUA has been able to alleviate for many. In fact, according to various studies, the success rate for this particular condition ranges from 75 to more than 96 percent.

Frozen Shoulder

The hallmark symptoms of a frozen shoulder are pain and either loss of motion or stiffness in the area. The pain is usually concentrated over the outer shoulder area. Sometimes it affects the upper arm as well.

But even more irritating than the pain, those who have this condition explain, is the inability to move the shoulder normally. Motion is even limited if another individual attempts to move the shoulder for you. Many individuals have found relief and restored range of motion from this condition through manipulation under anesthesia.

Stiff-Knee Syndrome

This serious condition, also known as arthrofibrosis, affects knee joints that have been either recently operated on or injured. Because of the traumatic event, either the surgery or the injury, internal scar tissue grows in the area around the knee. The growth of this tissue is then accompanied by a shrinking and subsequent tightening of the joint capsule. In some cases, even the neighboring tendons outside of the joint also become stiff.

This tightening process can continue, eventually causing severe restrictions to the motion of the leg. In some instances, individuals have been known to lose the ability to either fully straighten or bend their knee. This particular health condition very often responds poorly to conventional treatment. However, this type of condition responds well to manipulation under anesthesia. The manipulations literally release the scar tissue that is causing the restriction of movement.

Torticollis

This condition is a continual contraction of your neck muscles, which causes your head to turn to one side. You may know it by its alternative name: wryneck. If you have a family history of this problem, then you've probably developed it gradually over a number of years.

Some individuals, however, acquire it suddenly, usually from a trauma or, in some instances, as a result of an adverse reaction to certain medications. If you have this condition, MUA may be able to help correct it.

TMJ Disorders

If you suffer from this group of disorders involving the temporomandibular joint, you may find relief from manipulation under anesthesia. Your TMJ is the ball-and-socket joint on either side of your head, located in the area where your lower jawbone, the mandible, joins with the temporal bone of your skill.

Migraine Headaches

MUA may help you to end those excruciating migraine headaches, the type that can disrupt your activities and make you bedridden for a day...or more. If you suffer from migraines, then you know just how devastating this pain and its accompanying symptoms can be.

The medical community has studied this and has documented evidence. The Australian professional publication *International Journal of Headache* reported the results of a study in which five thousand individuals diagnosed with migraine headaches were treated with manipulation under anesthesia. Long-term follow-up on the group discovered that 90 percent of the individuals were still headache-free. And all it took was a three-day series of MUA followed with post-MUA therapy.

Many individuals find that the conservative, nonsurgical treatments have not alleviated their conditions. They then turn to MUA with great success. In fact, some individuals have suffered for a decade or more with migraine headaches that have been unresponsive to conservative care.

Before You Undergo MUA

Before recommending this procedure, most doctors will ensure that your particular condition doesn't respond to physical therapy or in-office manipulation. That's why your doctor may have you undergo a minimum of six weeks of conservative care involving in-office manipulation and physical therapy.

If, after six weeks of this type of care, you are still in considerable pain, then the topic of manipulation under anesthesia may be discussed.

Chapter 3:

How Your Doctor Determines If MUA Is Right for You

Candidates are selected for manipulation under anesthesia after obtaining an adequate history, thorough physical examination, the appropriate diagnostic imaging, and laboratory tests necessary for an accurate diagnosis of the underlying condition.

The first step is to provide your doctor with a full and accurate history of your health. Don't be shy. Tell your physician everything. This not only allows your doctor to get to know you and how your system works, but also gives him or her clues as to how well you will respond to the anesthesia.

Another reason for this detailed history is quite clear. Medical documentation must illustrate that you have pursued other types of treatments, without success, for your pain condition. Your doctor must have this information documented in order to perform this procedure.

Some aspects of your medical history that your doctor will be interested in documenting are the following:
- The presence of fibrosis or myofibrosis, the existing fibrous adhesions/scar tissue, in your affected area
- Supporting diagnostic testing indicating the cause of the pain
- Previous treatment, which have been non-responsive
- Lab work
- Physical exam including EKG

The Physical Examination

When your doctor performs the physical examination, he or she will be focusing particular attention on the affected joints and spine, as well as the other areas of concern. The doctor will palpate the spine and joints as well as visually view it for any abnormalities.

The doctor may inspect your skin to check if the sympathetic nervous system has produced any changes in the skin. The changes your doctor is searching for include, but are not limited to, swelling, the texture of the tissues, and temperature fluctuations in certain areas, as well as visual inspection and palpation of the skin. Typically, manifestation of sympathetic nervous system changes includes edema, tissue texture, increase or decrease of moisture, temperature changes, etc. Additionally, digital palpation identifies increased or decreased changes in muscle and fascia tone, which lead to altered biomechanics (i.e., does the affected area feel warmer than the rest of the body?). The doctor will evaluate the area to see if there's an increase or decrease in the amount of moisture.

Once your physical examination is completed, the doctor will then order the pertinent diagnostic tests necessary to complete the prerequisites for the MUA procedure. Your doctor will insist that you undergo certain laboratory examinations that will further evaluate your health. The purpose of these tests is two-fold: they substantiate a diagnosis that establishes you as a candidate for the MUA procedure and help to give your doctor a better view of your general health for purposes of undergoing the anesthesia.

What Types of Tests Are Involved?

Your doctor may choose any or all of the following tests described below. The intention of the following material is not to make you an expert on any of these tests. But, rather, when your doctor does refer to them, you will at least be familiar with a few of the terms, taking much of the mystery out of the language for you.

CBC Studies

While these tests are ominous-sounding, they really are nothing more than complete blood count tests that determine the make-up of your blood. For your part of this test, you need to do nothing more than give a blood sample.

A major section of the CBC is the measurement of the concentration of white blood cells and red blood cells, as well as the platelets in your blood. The blood work must be completed within thirty days of the procedure.

SMA 6

This is another type of blood test, normally referred to as a chemistry scan. This test, rather than measuring the number of blood cells, examines the chemical make-up of your blood. For example, some tests may examine the levels of electrolytes your blood contains. Your health care provider will want to obtain a profile of your blood's chemistry in order to get a picture of your complete health, not just your pain. Depending on what is found, your doctor will be able to tell you how your system will handle the light anesthesia and sedation.

X-Rays

If you are fifty years old or older, and/or a smoker, you will undergo a chest X-ray. This is extremely valuable in evaluating your heart as well as your chest wall, and will help to evaluate the state of your health as a candidate for the anesthetic. Depending on the location of your pain, your doctor may order X-rays on various joints of your body. This gives your doctor a better view of the extent of the problem.

In addition to X-rays, MRI scans, or CT scans, a musculoskeletal sonogram or nerve conduction velocity test may be ordered.

EKG

EKG stands for "electrocardiogram." It evaluates the electrical activity of your heart, which translates into line tracings on paper. Your doctor will want to make sure there is no hidden pathology with your heart that the anesthesia could affect.

Electrodiagnostic Tests

Electrodiagnostic studies of the appropriate spinal region should be performed to rule out specific neurological dysfunction. These tests confirm or differentiate diagnosis of neuropathy, radiculopathy, or plexopathy. They show the presence or lack of nerve compression, and localize and assess the degree of injury along the course of a nerve.

Contraindications for MUA

MUA is not an available option with some conditions, including:

- Pregnancy
- Excessive spinal osteoporosis
- Advanced heart disease
- Anyone over sixty-five years of age
- Bone-weakening diseases
- Cancer
- Certain circulatory diseases
- Uncontrolled diabetes
- Tuberculosis of the bone
- Fractures
- Acute arthritis
- Acute gout
- Syphilitic articular or periarticular lesions
- Gonorrheal spinal arthritis
- Evidence of cord or caudal compression by tumor, ankylosis, and malacia bone disease

Chapter 4:

෬∾෧

Specific Techniques of MUA

The specific techniques your health care practitioner uses during manipulation under anesthesia largely depend on the location of your specific pain, the severity of the pain, and your individualized symptoms.

The doctor's goal is essentially the same as in providing you with an in-office manipulation. That is to decrease or eliminate the pain and provide you with a broader range of motion in regards to the function of your body.

While you are fully conscious in the doctor's office, the typical or standard manipulation is usually described as being "high-velocity/low-amplitude thrust" or impulse. Your doctor uses this specific motion in order to overcome your system's protective reflex mechanism.

This protective mechanism works to prevent the separation and movement of the joints. During joint manipulation, the movement extends beyond the entire passive range of motion and beyond the elastic barrier.

Beyond this barrier lies what, in medical terms, is referred to as the paraphysiological space. This is where joint "cavitation" occurs. In essence, cavitation is the "popping" sound most people think of when they envision manipulation.

The Low-Velocity/High-Amplitude Technique of MUA

The techniques used in MUA are best described as "low-velocity/high-amplitude thrusts." The thrusting force used is carefully applied, considering the natural resistance of the injury to therapy. Because you are under the influence of mild sedation, your body allows for more joint movement than what can occur during a normal in-office session.

The goal of applying these thrusts is to have the force of the movement pass through the muscle tone to stretch and lengthen the shortened muscle beyond its normal active range. Then the targeted areas of the spine or extremity can be moved through to the passive range, where the doctor would be able to feel the resistance of the fibrotic scar tissue.

Your doctor continues to carefully manipulate the subject areas until the elastic barrier has been reached, an event that had been elusive during the in-office sessions. Your doctor applies consistent low-velocity/high-amplitude movement into that paraphysiological space with postural kinesthetic maneuvers.

Techniques utilized under anesthesia may vary from patient to patient, depending on the involved tissues and existing relative contraindications and/or possible complications that may exist. Some of the techniques include:

> **Soft-tissue procedures**—lateral stretching, linear stretching, deep pressure, traction, and/or separation of muscle origin and insertion
>
> Tissue: periarticular
> Goals: decrease muscle spasm and increase tissue mobility
>
> **Articulatory procedures** (*mobilization without impulse, low-velocity techniques*)—placing articulation through full anatomic range of motion. A passive, serial, repetitive, oscillatory rhythmic springing force in the direction of restriction is performed.

Tissue: periarticular and articular
Goals: increase quantity of motion-gradual movement
of restrictive barrier to restore range of motion;
increase quality of motion and smooth range of
movement with normal elasticity and feel

Specific joint mobilization procedure—mobilization with impulse, high-velocity technique. The extrinsic operator applies thrust, overcoming restrictive articular movement. Engagement of the restrictive barrier and thrust through the barrier occurs and achieves normal joint movement.

Tissue: articular and intra-articular
Goals: increase of joint angle of motion to reduce joint
restrictions; reduction of hypertonicity; stretch
shortened, fibrosed connective tissues of the
articulation

It is at this point that the cavitation of the joint occurs. Your chiropractor may describe this as "releasing" your joint. While this is the goal for which the doctor has been hoping, the job isn't quite finished yet. The chiropractic doctor will still continue exerting small amounts of force to stretch, lengthen, and dissolve the adhesions and fibrosis, which originally created the pain and limited movement.

In a full spinal procedure, your physician will apply techniques especially designed for MUA. Your doctor will start in the cervical spine, which begins at the base of the skull. At the cervical spine, the doctor may gently stretch the spinal area as well as gently bend the head forward and to either side.

From there, the doctor moves to the thoracic spine. This section of the spinal column is located directly below the cervical section in the chest area. The thoracic spine contains a total of twelve vertebrae, and connects to the ribs. One of its many tasks is to protect the vital organs.

Finally, the doctor moves to the lumbar area, the lower section of your spine, and performs similar techniques. The doctor will gently stretch and lengthen this area. Additionally, he or she may massage this area and place your body through some knee-to-chest rolls. The joints that are applicable will be mobilized and stretched next.

More Techniques

Your doctor may also choose to perform procedures aimed at the soft tissues. In this case, the physician will induce a series of lateral stretches, side to side, as well as applying deep pressure to the specific areas affected. The doctor may also provide traction in order to stretch and lengthen the affected muscles. The goals of these soft-tissue procedures are to decrease muscle spasms and increase mobility of the tissues.

Among other techniques, your doctor may choose methods known as articulatory procedures. These are the low-velocity techniques discussed earlier used to increase the range of motion in the spine and joints.

Depending on your condition, your doctor may choose to use several high-velocity techniques on specific areas. This is known as specific joint mobilization procedure. The doctor will manipulate the area with the specific purpose of overcoming the restrictive movement until normal movement of the joint can be achieved through manipulation. The goal of this procedure is to reduce the restrictive movement of the joint and increase its range of motion. This also helps to stretch and lengthen the shortened connective tissue affected by the scar tissue.

Of course, the overriding and underlying purpose of all of these techniques or procedures is to ultimately eliminate the pain as much as possible and to perform the biomechanical changes that last.

Chapter 5:

∽

Post-Procedure:
The Therapy after the MUA Is Critical!

What happens after MUA? In one word: relief.

After undergoing the MUA procedure, you will experience your range of motion restored at the treated areas. Most individuals who undergo MUA are more than pleased with their new-found range of motion, even though there is usually some temporarily added muscle soreness similar to the feeling of having completed an aggressive exercise routine. In cases involving symptoms caused by disturbance from adhesions and shortened tissues, there should be a significant change, either immediately or within a short period of time following the procedures.

Not only that, but you will also realize that the pain you have been living with for so long is significantly decreased, and, in some instances, completely gone.

It is not unusual to experience some temporary soreness in the muscles and possible bruising (which resolves within a week or two) after the procedure. Again, you may feel as if you have been exercising vigorously.

Once you have successfully completed the outpatient portion of the MUA, the follow-up visits and procedures begin. There's still work to be accomplished to ensure that you heal properly and that the results last.

How you treat your condition after you've undergone manipulation under anesthesia is vitally important to your recovery. You should begin this important care soon after the procedure is completed. In fact, what you do to take care of your condition could mean the ultimate success or failure of your procedure.

Dr. I.C. Rumney emphasizes this point in the *Journal of the American Osteopathic Association.* He writes:

> *Even after the manipulative procedures release the fibrosis, one must institute an adequate program of physical therapy and exercise. If one does not prevent, or lessen, the formation of fibrous tissue, the patient's original problem will recur.*

The post-procedure therapy involves approximately six to eight weeks of intensive therapy, all of which occurs in your doctor's office. For the most part, your doctor will perform similar stretches and adjustments that were performed during the MUA.

Basically, the goals of the after-care program include:

- Caring for any lingering inflammation
- Ensuring that your free, uninterrupted movements of the spinal joints and muscles continue
- Providing for the proper healing of the affected area
- Strengthening of the muscles that have been affected and not used with any frequency
- Ensuring, as much as possible, that there is no reformation of the adhesions that originally caused your pain

Normally, your doctor will have you complete a combination of stretching and flexibility exercises as well as exercises aimed at strengthening the subject areas.

In the doctor's attempt to minimize the reformation of the adhesions that caused your original pain, passive manipulations and active exercises are prescribed. Your doctor may also have you go through additional therapies such as:

- Electrical muscle stimulation (EMS)
- Ultrasound
- Hot moist packs
- Massage

Electrical muscle stimulation, also known by its abbreviation, EMS, is a form of therapy that aims at strengthening muscles that haven't been used for some time. EMS helps the muscles gain strength faster than on their own—the same muscles that you have avoided using for so long because of the pain.

Your doctor may prescribe ultrasound for you. The purpose of this therapy is to help relieve any muscle spasms. Ultrasound therapy makes use of high- and low-frequency sound waves to penetrate into the muscle. The end result is a warming of your muscle, which promotes tissue relaxation. Ultrasound treatment also helps to increase blood circulation in the affected area, which, in the long run, aids in the healing of the muscle. Ultrasound can also be used to decrease inflammation.

Massage therapy may also be administered for the affected area. This helps to restore blood flow as well as to relax tight muscles.

Your doctor may also prescribe cryotherapy, which involves placing an ice pack on the affected area. Ice is a great therapeutic tool; first and foremost, it reduces inflammation. Since inflammation is the cause of pain, you can be confident that this will also help to relieve any residual pain either due to the manipulation or released muscles that are in the process of healing.

Therapeutic exercises, such as stretching and strengthening of the affected areas, will also be administered. Spinal adjustments are commonly performed to help restore and maintain the proper biomechanics implemented during the MUA procedure. This regimented post-MUA therapy will help the patient regain pre-condition strength and help prevent future pain and disability.

෨

Conclusion

With sixty years of history and a myriad of favorable studies to support the MUA procedure, manipulation under anesthesia appears to be a viable, effective alternative for individuals who experience stubborn, chronic pain.

While the MUA procedure may sound like major surgery, it couldn't be farther from that. MUA is a technique that allows your doctor to perform a much more thorough series of manipulative maneuvers while you are lightly sedated and under a mild anesthesia. These maneuvers help to ease the pain and increase the range of motion in the area affected by discomfort and stiffness.

MUA is extremely successful on such conditions as:

- Neck and back pain
- Sciatica
- Neuralgia
- Radiculitis
- Headache/migraine headache
- TMJ (Costen's syndrome)
- Curvature of the spine
- Joint calcifications
- Disc herniations/bulges
- Frozen shoulder
- Fibromyalgia
- Myofascitis
- Capsulitis of the hip
- Torticollis
- Carpal tunnel syndrome
- Piriformis syndrome
- Pelvic instability

- Gait abnormality/imbalance
- Stiff-knee syndrome

Much of its success lies in the fact that the greater extent of manipulation dissolves scar tissues inside the joints and muscles, as well as any fibrous adhesions that have formed due to injury or micro-trauma.

There are many advantages to the MUA procedure; however, there is one drawback. To be eligible for MUA, the patient must have exhausted most forms of conservative therapy, which means a minimum of six to eight weeks of failed conservative treatment. MUA is used when most forms of conservative treatment have failed, and, in some cases, when back surgery failed.

For a period of time, MUA procedures were not widely utilized because of the available anesthetics. But the advent of intravenous sedation use has spurred an MUA renaissance. Due to the high success rate for patients who had previously experienced chronic pain, MUA procedures are now covered by most major insurance plans.

In my experience with MUA, I have seen patients who have suffered needlessly with poor quality of life and were in constant pain. After completing the two-month program (including eight weeks of post-therapy), 90 percent of our patients have been able to return to their normal lives. It's amazing what healthy people take for granted, such as sitting on the toilet, going for a walk in the park, standing, and sleeping. When pain robs you of normal function, it robs you of your spirit. MUA brings people back to life!

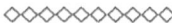

Patient Testimonials

Here's what some of Dr. Morgen's patients have to say:

"I have had chronic back, hip, feet, and neck pain for years. After receiving MUA, I have had an 80 percent overall improvement. It was not only a physically changing experience, but has improved my mental condition as well. I am now a much healthier and happier person. Thanks, Dr. Morgen." J.P.

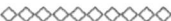

"When I was diagnosed with fibromyalgia, I was devastated. My neck and shoulder caused me severe pain and restricted range of motion. After receiving the MUA, my stiffness and range of motion improved significantly. I would highly recommend it to anyone diagnosed with fibromyalgia." S.S.

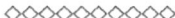

"I've had lower back pain for over twenty years and had difficulty performing simple tasks such as dusting, vacuuming, and bending over to tie shoes. Now I can perform all these tasks with no pain. Thank you, Dr. Morgen and your assisting doctors. You knew what I needed." V.R.

"Since receiving the MUA procedure, I have noticed a significant decrease in my pains from fibromyalgia. My range of motion is so much better. I can perform simple tasks around the house such as dusting without being 'wiped out.' I also have a significant decrease in the number of headaches since the MUA. Thank you." C.M.

◇◇◇◇◇◇◇◇◇◇

"I have been suffering from headaches since the past five years almost daily, migraines twice per month, and had lower back pain since eighteen years. After having had the MUA procedure, my lower back pain is GONE! I can now stand on my feet for over eight hours, bend over and touch the ground, and twist side to side without the pain. Headaches have disappeared! All this without drugs, amazing! Thank you for your wonderful care and concern." E.Y.

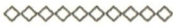

"Before having the MUA, I was taking four to five Vicodins per day just to be able to get up and walk. Within three weeks after the MUA, I am completely off all the pain medications and feeling so much better. I was also surprised that the anesthesia I received had no side effects and I awoke within ten minutes. I am so glad that I chose this over pain management and back surgery. Thanks again." R.W.

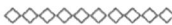

"Working as a lineman for FPL, my job can be extremely physical, especially on my lower back. I had always felt stiff and not very flexible, but with the MUA, I have noticed a significant increase in my flexibility. Just doing simple tasks at work, like bending down and picking something up, I'm not struggling with the stiffness that I had become so accustomed to. My flexibility has increased by at least 50 percent since receiving the MUA. Now I can touch my toes and don't have the constant pain." P.T.

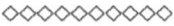

"As a truck driver, I was diagnosed with frozen shoulder and had severe difficulty lifting my arm, driving, and washing my hair. I was concerned I would lose all function, so after receiving the MUA, my range of motion and activities were fully restored. I am thrilled. Thank you." D.J.

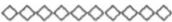

"I was sick and tired of the constant pain I always felt. It consumed me, made me exhausted, and was taking over my life. After being accepted as a candidate for the MUA and having the procedure performed, I thank God I no longer live in constant pain 24/7 and can sleep through the night. I no longer wince with every step I take. I am now pain-free and am eternally grateful. Thank you, Dr. M." P.J.

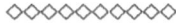

"For many years, I have suffered from neck pain with numbness and tingling in my arms and fingertips, making it difficult to perform daily activities. I was very skeptical of the MUA. Since undergoing the procedure, I have regained the feeling in my arms and have excellent mobility in my neck. I feel like myself again. I would highly recommend this procedure for those suffering with chronic pain." T.M.

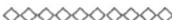

"Prior to the MUA, I had numbness and tingling in my left leg due to a disc herniation. After receiving the MUA, the numbness and tingling has subsided. My lower back pain has improved 95 percent. This procedure was a life-saver." J.Z.

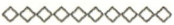

❧

Case Studies

Manipulation under Anesthesia (MUA) Gives Significant Relief to a Patient Diagnosed with Fibromyalgia Syndrome (FMS)

A Case Study:

A forty-two-year-old Caucasian female presented to my office four weeks ago with severe chronic neck, mid- to low-back pain, bilateral shoulder, leg, and hip pain, headaches, numbness in her right hand and right foot, and extreme fatigue. She worked as an RN at an outpatient center. Her pain began five years ago and she was recently diagnosed with FMS, as her symptoms were progressively getting worse in the last three years. Her activities of daily living (ADLs) included difficulty with prolonged sitting, standing, and sleeping, and inability to exercise and lift her right arm to comb her hair. She also had difficulty driving to see her patients. Examination revealed fibrous adhesions with tautness and shortening of the hamstrings, quadriceps, tensor fascia lata, and piriformis muscles bilaterally (both sides). Restricted Range of Motion (ROM) was noted in the cervical and lumbosacral regions by more than 50 percent. The pain was dull, constant, and rated an eight to ten out of ten on the Visual Analog Scale (VAS) with respect to all of her symptoms noted above; ten is the worst level of pain. Upper extremity (UE) dermatomes sensation revealed hypoesthesia (less sensation) C6 on the right, and lower extremity (LE) dermatomes revealed hypoesthesia L5 on the right. UE and LE reflexes were within normal limits (WNL). UE and LE manual muscle testing revealed +5 bilaterally. The pain had progressively become worse in the last three months and she wanted a non-drug, non-invasive solution.

Diagnostic imaging: Due to the patient's clinical and exam findings, a lumbar spine MRI without contrast was ordered by her M.D. The lumbar spine MRI revealed the following: disc bulging at L3-L4, L4-L5.

Recommended course of treatment: three consecutive days of manipulation under anesthesia (MUA) followed by a six- week intensive physical therapy program.

Conclusion: After receiving three consecutive days of MUA performed at an outpatient surgical center, the patient noticed an 85 percent improvement of her symptoms. The fatigue has sub-sided, her ROM has increased in her cervical, lumbar, right shoul-der, and LE muscles bilaterally, and she can now resume her activi-ties without difficulty. The ROM in her hamstrings, TFL (Tensor Fasciae Latae), quadriceps, and piriformis muscles bilaterally has improved by more than 60 percent. Her pain is rated a two out of ten on the VAS. She has reached her goals of increasing her mobil-ity, and reducing her fatigue and pain levels. The patient is excited to resume her normal activities with full function and without a dependency on invasive measures.

Manipulation under Anesthesia (MUA) on a Patient Diagnosed with Chronic Low-Back Pain and HNP (Disc Herniation) of C4-C5

A Case Study:

A fifty-eight-year-old Caucasian female presented to my office two months ago with moderate to severe chronic neck and low-back pain with no known onset of injury. She worked as an engineer, sitting at a desk all day. Her activities included difficulty turning her neck, sleeping, walking, and sitting for prolonged periods of time. Examination revealed scoliosis in the thoracolumbar spine and restricted ROM in her cervical and lumbar regions. The pain was rated a nine to ten out of ten on the VAS in the cervical and lumbar areas. LE reflexes and dermatomes were normal. UE reflexes were WNL, and UE dermatomes revealed a +1 DTR (decreased reflex) at C5 on the left. The pain had progressively become worse in the last three months and she had exhausted conservative management.

Recommended course of treatment: three consecutive days of manipulation under anesthesia (MUA) followed by a six-week intensive physical therapy program.

Conclusion: After receiving three consecutive days of MUA performed at an outpatient surgical center, the patient noticed an 85 percent improvement of her symptoms. She can now resume her ADLs without difficulty. Her ROM is full in the cervical and lumbar spine. Her pain is rated a 1.5 to two out of ten on the VAS. The patient is excited to resume her normal ADLs with full function and without a dependency on invasive measures.

Manipulation under Anesthesia (MUA) on a Patient Diagnosed with Chronic Low-Back Pain and Multi-Level HNP of the Lumbar Spine

A Case Study:

A fifty-six-year-old Caucasian female presented to my office with moderate chronic lower back pain, which began twenty years ago with no known onset of injury. She worked thirty years as a postal worker, but sat at a desk all day. Her activities included difficulty turning, bending, sleeping, walking, and sitting for prolonged periods of time. Examination revealed shortening of the hamstrings, piriformis, and erector spinae muscles bilaterally, and restricted ROM in the thoracolumbar region. The pain was rated as an eight out of ten on the VAS in the lumbar region. LE reflexes and dermatomes were normal. The pain had progressively become worse in the last two years and she was tired of it.

Diagnostic studies: A lumbar MRI without contrast was ordered and revealed a disc herniation at T11-T12, T12-L1, L1-L2, and disc bulging at L3-L4 and L4-L5.

Recommended course of treatment: three consecutive days of manipulation under anesthesia (MUA) followed by a six-week intensive physical therapy program.

Conclusion: After receiving three consecutive days of MUA performed at an outpatient surgical center, the patient noticed a 65 percent improvement of her symptoms. She can now resume her activities without difficulty, which include household chores and sleeping through the night without waking due to pain. Her ROM is full in the thoracolumbar spine. Her pain is rated a three out of ten on the VAS. The patient is excited to resume her normal activities with full function and without a dependency on invasive measures.

Manipulation under Anesthesia (MUA) on a Patient Diagnosed with Chronic Pain, Lumbar Disc Herniations, and Cervical Radiculopathy

A Case Study:

A thirty-six-year-old Caucasian male presented to my office one month ago with moderate to severe chronic neck and low-back pain, and numbness in his arms and hands bilaterally, with no known onset of injury. He worked as a lineman for Florida Power and Light, utilizing his hands most of the day. The pain began sixteen years ago. He had failed epidural and cortisone injection therapy. His activities included difficulty turning his neck, sleeping, walking, and sitting for prolonged periods of time. Examination revealed multiple trigger points and fibrous adhesions proximal to the cervical, thoracic, and lumbosacral spine, and restricted ROM in his cervical and lumbar regions. The pain was rated an eight to ten out of ten on the VAS in the cervical and lumbar areas. LE reflexes and dermatomes were normal. UE reflexes were normal, and UE dermatomes revealed hypoesthesia (less sensation) at C6-C8 on the right. The pain had progressively become worse in the last three months and he had exhausted conservative management.

Diagnostic studies: A cervical and lumbar MRI were ordered and revealed disc bulging at C5-C6, C6-C7, and L3-L4, and HNP at L4-L5 and L5-S1.

Recommended course of treatment: three consecutive days of manipulation under anesthesia (MUA) followed by a six-week intensive physical therapy program.

Conclusion: After receiving three consecutive days of MUA performed at an outpatient surgical center, the patient noticed a 95 percent improvement of his symptoms. The numbness in his arms and hands has subsided, and the discomfort in his neck and back are minimal. He can now resume his activities without difficulty, which include sleeping without waking due to numbness, prolonged sitting and standing without pain, and full range of motion in his cervical and lumbar spine. His pain is rated a one to two out of ten on the VAS. The patient is excited to resume his normal activities with full function and without a dependency on invasive measures.

Manipulation under Anesthesia (MUA) Performed on a Patient Diagnosed with Spinal Stenosis C5-C6, Post-Surgical Lumbago, and Bilateral Plantarfasciitis

A Case Study:

A forty-nine-year-old Caucasian male presented to my office with moderately severe chronic neck pain, which began over ten years ago with no known onset of injury, chronic bilateral plantarfasciitis, which began more than five years ago, and post-surgical lumbago from fifteen years ago. He worked in construction. His activities included difficulty turning, bending, sleeping, and walking, and sitting and standing for prolonged periods of time. Examination revealed shortening of the suboccipitals, upper trapezius, levator scapulae, scalene, hamstrings, piriformis, erector spinae, and plantarfascia muscles bilaterally. Restricted ROM was noted in the cervical and lumbar region. The pain was rated as an eight to nine out of ten on the VAS in the cervical and lumbar region and in his feet. UE and LE reflexes and dermatomes were normal. The pain had progressively become worse in the last two years and he was tired of it.

Diagnostic studies: A cervical MRI without contrast was ordered and revealed mild spinal stenosis at C5-C6.

Recommended course of treatment: three consecutive days of manipulation under anesthesia (MUA) followed by an eight-week intensive physical therapy program.

Conclusion: After receiving three consecutive days of MUA performed at an outpatient surgical center, the patient noticed an 80 percent improvement of his symptoms. He can now resume his ADLs without difficulty, which include bending, sitting, standing, and sleeping through the night without waking due to pain. His cervical ROM has marked improvement. His pain is rated a two out of ten on the VAS. The patient is excited to resume his normal activities with full function and without a dependency on invasive measures.

༄

Research Studies

Scientific Evaluation of MUA

Multiple prospective and retrospective clinical studies have been performed evaluating MUA in chronic unresolved back pain, acute and chronic disc herniations, cervicogenic cephalgia, and many other neuromusculoskeletal conditions with attendant articular dyskinesia.

Robert Mensor, M.D., orthopedic surgeon, compared the outcomes of MUA and laminectomy (back surgery) in patients with lumbar intervertebral disc lesions and found that 83 percent of MUA patients had good to excellent results, while only 51 percent of the surgical patients reported the same outcome.

Donald Chrisman, M.D., orthopedic surgeon, reported that 51 percent of patients with unequivocal disc lesions and unrelieved symptoms, after conservative care had been rendered, reported good to excellent results post-MUA at a three-year follow-up.[1]

Bradford & Siehl reported on seven hundred and twenty-three MUA patients, the largest clinical trial conducted on MUA procedures, and found that 71 percent had good results, 25 percent had fair results, and 4 percent ultimately required surgical intervention.[2]

Krumhansl and Nowacek reported on one hundred and seventy-one patients who experienced constant intractable pain, of durations from several months to eighteen years, and who underwent MUA. All patients had failed at previous conservative interventions. Results reported that, post-MUA, 25 percent had no pain at all and were "cured"; 50 percent were "much improved" with pain markedly reduced and ADLs essentially unaffected; 20 percent were "better, but" pain continued to interfere with activities; and, finally, 5 percent had minimal or no relief.[3]

West, et al, reported in a 1998 study of one hundred and seventy-seven patients that 68.6 percent of those out of work returned to unrestricted work activities after a series of three consecutive MUA procedures at six months post-MUA, that 58.4 percent of the MUA patients receiving medications prior to the procedure required no prescription medication post-procedure, and, finally, that 60.1 percent of patients with lumbar pain resolved it with post-MUA series of procedures.[4]

In 2002, Palmieri, et al, demonstrated the clinical efficacy of MUA performed in a series of three consecutive procedures. The average Numeric Pain Scale scores in the MUA group decreased by 50 percent, and the average Roland-Morris Questionnaire scores decreased by 51 percent compared to the control group (a decreased score signifies improvements).

In addition to the extensive literature, there are currently ongoing prospective clinical trials with appropriate outcome instruments assessing the clinical and fiscal efficacy of MUA in a selected patient population.

The medical literature is replete with case studies and literature reviews on MUA, in addition to clinical trials, all of which report positive outcomes. Further research is ongoing. It is important to note that, to date, there has been no clinical trial that demonstrates MUA to be ineffective in an appropriately selected patient population.

Reference Notes

1. Chrisman, O.D., et al, "A study of the results following rotary manipulation of the lumbar intervertebral disc syndrome," *J Bone Joint Surg,* 1964: 46-A: 517

2. Siehl, D., Bradford, W. (1952), "Manipulation of the low back under general anesthesia," *J Am Osteopath Assoc* 52 (4): 239-42, P M I D 13011132

3. Krumhansl, B.R., Nowacek, C.J., "Manipulation under anesthesia," *Modern manual therapy of the vertebral column,* Edinburgh: Churchill Livingstone, 1986

4. West, D.C., C.C.R.D., Mathews, M.D., Miller, PA-C, Kent, M.D., "Effect of Management of Spinal Pain in 200 Patients Evaluated for Manipulation Under Anesthesia," *J. Neurol Orthop Med Surg* (1998), 18: pp. 31-42

∽

Supporting Studies

There are several research studies about the effectiveness of manipulation under anesthesia, including:

83 percent of 600 patients with EMG-verified radiculopathies reported significant improvement (Robert Mensor, M.D.).

Patients who had back pain for a minimum of ten years reported an 87 percent recovery rate after MUA (1987, Ongly, et al).

Fifty-one percent of patients with resolved symptoms reported good to excellent results three years post-MUA (Donald Chrisman, M.D.).

Seventy-one percent of seven hundred and twenty-three MUA patients had good results (returned to normal activity relatively symptom-free) and 25.3 percent had fair results (returned to normal activity with slight residuals), and that flexibility, elasticity, and range of motion can be restored following MUA (Bradford and Siehl).

Eighty-three percent of five hundred and seventeen patients treated with MUA responded well (Paul Kuo, M.D., professor of orthopedic surgery).

The medical literature demonstrates that for over forty years, chronic neuromuscular skeletal conditions that have failed with the conservative protocol respond well to manipulation under anesthesia.

The overall effectiveness of spinal manipulation under anesthesia has been reported by researchers, with success rates varying according to case selection criteria.

Diagnoses of herniated discs reported excellent to good results in:

Sixty percent (P.C. Colonna and Z.B. Friendenberg, 1949)

Sixty-four percent (Merrill C. Mensor, M.D., 1949)

Sixty percent (Donald Sielh, D.C., 1963)

Diagnoses of myofibrositis reported excellent to good results in:
96.3 percent (Donald Siehl, O.D., 1963)
Seventy-five percent (B.R. Krumhansi and C.J. Nowacek, 1988)

∽

References

1. Greenman, P.E.: "Manipulation with the patient under anesthesia," *J. Amer. Osteopathic Assoc.*, 92(9):1159 -1167, Sept. 1992

2. West, D.C., C.C.R.D., Mathews, M.D., Miller, PA-C, Kent, M.D., "Effect of Management of Spinal Pain in 200 Patients Evaluated for Manipulation Under Anesthesia," *J. Neurol Orthop Med Surg* (1998), 18: pp. 31-42

3. "Guidelines for Chiropractic Quality Assurance and Practice Parameters: Proceedings of the Mercy Center Consensus Conference, Burlingame, CA, January 25-30, 1992," S. Haldeman, et al (eds.), Gaithersburg, MD: Aspen Publishers, Inc. 1993

4. Dreyfuss, P., et al, "MUJA: Manipulation under joint anesthesia/analgesia: A treatment approach for recalcitrant low back pain of synovial joint origin," *J Manipulative Physiol Ther*, 1995, 18:537-546

5. Davis, C.G., "Chronic cervical spine pain treated with manipulation under anesthesia," *J Neuromusculoskeletal Syst*, 1996, 4:102-115

6. Francis, R., "Spinal manipulation under general anesthesia: A chiropractic approach in a hospital setting," *J Am Chiro Assoc.*, 1989, Dec: 39-41

7. Alexander, G.K., "Manipulation under anesthesia of lumbar post-laminectomy syndrome patients with epidural fibrosis and recurrent HNP," *J Am Chiro Assoc.*, 1993, June: 79-81

8. Hughes, B.L., "Management of cervical disk syndrome utilizing manipulation under anesthesia," *J Manipulative Physiol Ther*, 1993, 16:174-181

9. Aspegren, D.D., et al, "Manipulation under epidural anesthesia with corticosteroid injection: Two case reports," *J Manipulative Physiol Ther*, 1997, 20(9): 618-621

᚛

Physicians' Quotes

Here's what some physicians have to say about the MUA procedure:

"In my experience, I have had success with manipulation under anesthesia for the shoulder for conditions of adhesive capsulitis that occurs post-operatively and idiopathically. I would recommend a manipulation under anesthesia for the shoulder for specific conditions because of its low risk when performed by an experienced practitioner."

—Rena R. Amro, M.D., FAAOS, FACS
Diplomate, American Board of Orthopedic Surgery
Board Certified in Orthopaedic Surgery
Fellow, American Academy of Orthopedic Surgery
Fellow, American College of Surgeons
President, Palm Orthopaedic Institute, Inc.

"Having performed over one thousand MUA procedures since January 2007, it is truly remarkable seeing those patients feel and function better in their daily activities, their work, and their recreation. Listening to someone explain that they can now wash their car, lift their kids, and exercise longer without the pain level that they once had is very rewarding as a physician. I have seen great patient outcomes due to MUA, with our centers establishing an approximate 75 percent success rate of reduced or eliminated pain and improved quality of life."

—Steven Cimerberg, D.O., F.A.C.O.F.P
President, American College of Osteopathic Family Physicians
Broward County Osteopathic Medical Association
Past President, Nova Southeastern College of Osteopathic
Medicine Alumni
www.lipocenterofsouthflorida.com

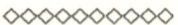

"I was amazed at the recovery rate and reduction in pain from day one to day three of the procedure. From my personal involvement in over one thousand MUAs, I would estimate an initial success rate of 80 to 85 percent. Our surgical team always explains to patients, however, an MUA is only the beginning of the healing process. Patients must continue with physical therapy for at least six to eight weeks post-surgery to receive the full benefits of MUA."

—Todd R. Zusmer, D.O.
Board Certified in Family Medicine
Osteopathic Manipulative Medicine

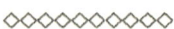

"Having treated patients over the past twenty-five years primarily for neuro-musculoskeletal pain and chronic pain syndromes, I was optimistic regarding the MUA procedure based on its theory and reports from my colleagues in both the medical and chiropractic fields. Now, having done a few hundred of these procedures myself, my expectations have been far exceeded and I have found the outcomes on my patients to be exceptional."

—Robert J. Mann, D.C.
Chiropractic Physician
COO of Universal Medical Concepts

"Since beginning performing manipulation under anesthesia, I have been gratified by the positive experience my patients have achieved by having the procedure done. Many have returned to my office months after the procedure saying how their lives have changed, returning them to the lifestyle that they had missed for so long due to chronic pain. We have impacted those with chronic daily headache, fibromyalgia, and sciatica, to name a few pain syndromes that we have treated with success. I can easily recommend this procedure for any patient suffering from a chronic pain syndrome."

—Michael A. Flicker, D.O.
Board Certified in Family Medicine
Osteopathic Manipulative Medicine
Associate Professor, Nova Southeastern

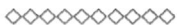

"Like most allopathic Western doctors, I was trained to treat chronic back pain using a specific algorithm. According to that plan, when the traditional combinations of 'conservative care' methods and medications have failed, I moved to other methods, such as: physical therapy, standard chiropractic manipulations, acupuncture, pain medicine injections, and others. Thereafter, many of my patients who were still suffering have moved to more permanent and risky options, such as major surgeries and rhizotomies, whenever those methods were deemed appropriate. Unfortunately, I often have patients who have exhausted this usual algorithm, but are still suffering from a debilitating level of pain and spasm. For such patients, manipulation under anesthesia (MUA), as performed by Dr. Morgen, has repeatedly proved to be a great new option—and sometimes even a godsend. One patient was helped so much by the procedure that she told me, 'Finally, something has given me back my life... I feel as if I can now start over after losing several years!'"

—Ronald M. Gazze, M.D.
Medical Director of FPL (Florida Power & Light)
Diplomate of the American Board of Family Medicine

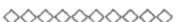

"I have recommended a few patients that have benefited from the MUA procedure. I feel that it's a great alternative for those patients that have chronic pain and those that want to avoid/delay a surgical procedure."
—Pedro Nam, M.D.
Diplomate Internal Medicine

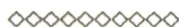

"I have had patients that had persistent pain despite aggressive medical therapy. After undergoing MUA, their pain was much improved. I am truly impressed."

—Michael J. Sinclair, M.D., F.A.A.F.P.
Board Certified Family Practice
Former Chairman, Department of Family Practice
Former Chief of Staff, Palms West Hospital
www.epilution.com

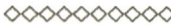

"When I first started doing anesthesia for MUA, I was a bit skeptical that this would relieve some patients' pain. I was amazed at how well it worked and how much their range of motion had improved. I've run into patients on the street several months later to find they still had pain relief. Another benefit was that these patients were able to decrease the amount of narcotics they were taking, allowing them to improve their quality of life."

—Thomas Hernandez, M.D.
Staff Anesthesiologist
Jupiter Medical Center

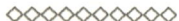

www.ingramcontent.com/pod-product-compliance
Lightning Source LLC
Chambersburg PA
CBHW020402290526
45785CB00005B/2408